Mediterranean Main Courses Cookbook

Enjoy your Dinner and your Lunch with 50 Delicious Main Courses Recipes

Carlo Montesanti

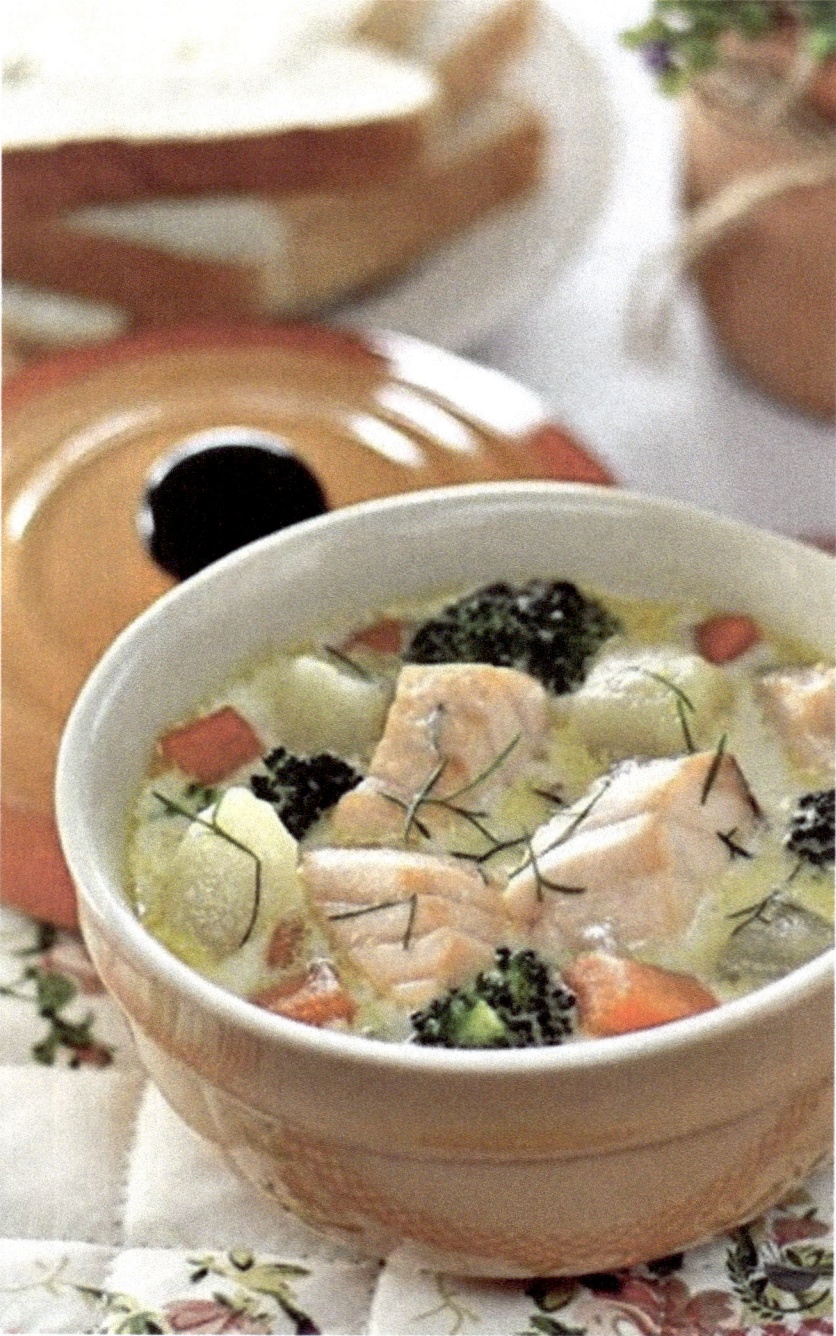

Table of Contents

Fish and Veggie Stew

Prep Time: 10 min

Cook Time: 1 h 30 min

Serve: 4

Ingredients:

- 6 lemon wedges, pulp separated and chopped and some of the peel reserved
- 2 tbsp. parsley, chopped
- 2 tomatoes, cut in halves, peeled and grated
- 2 tbsp. cilantro, chopped
- 2 garlic cloves, minced
- ½ tsp. paprika
- 2 tbsp. water
- ½ cup water
- ½ tsp. cumin, ground
- Salt and black pepper to taste

- 4 bass fillets

- ¼ cup olive oil

- 3 carrots, sliced

- 1 red bell pepper, sliced lengthwise and thinly cut in strips

- 1 and ¼ lb. potatoes, peeled and sliced

- ½ cup olives

- 1 red onion, thinly sliced

Preparation:

1. In a bowl, mix tomatoes with lemon pulp, cilantro, parsley, cumin, garlic, paprika, salt, pepper, 2 tbsp. water, 2 tsp. oil and the fish, toss to coat and keep in the fridge for 30 minutes. Heat a saucepan with the water and some salt over medium high heat, add potatoes and carrots, stir, cook for 10 minutes and drain.

2. Heat a pan over medium heat, add bell pepper and ¼ cup water, cover, cook for 5 minutes and take off heat.

3. Coat a saucepan with remaining oil, add potatoes and carrots, ¼ cup water, onion slices, fish and its marinade,

bell pepper strips, olives, salt and pepper, toss gently, cook for 45 minutes, divide into bowls and serve.

Tomato Soup

Prep Time: 60 min

Cook Time: 2 min

Serve: 4

Ingredients:

- ½ green bell pepper, chopped
- ½ red bell pepper, chopped
- 1 and ¾ lb. tomatoes, chopped
- ¼ cup bread, torn
- 9 tbsp. extra virgin olive oil
- 1 garlic clove, minced
- 2 tsp. sherry vinegar
- Salt and black pepper to taste
- 1 tbsp. cilantro, chopped
- A pinch of cumin, ground

Preparation:

1. In a blender, mix green and red bell peppers with tomatoes, salt, pepper, 6 tbsp. oil, and the other ingredients except the bread and cilantro, and pulse well. Keep in the fridge for 1 hour.

2. Heat a pan with remaining oil over medium high heat, add bread pieces, and toast them for 1 minute.

3. Divide cold soup into bowls, top with bread cubes and cilantro then serve.

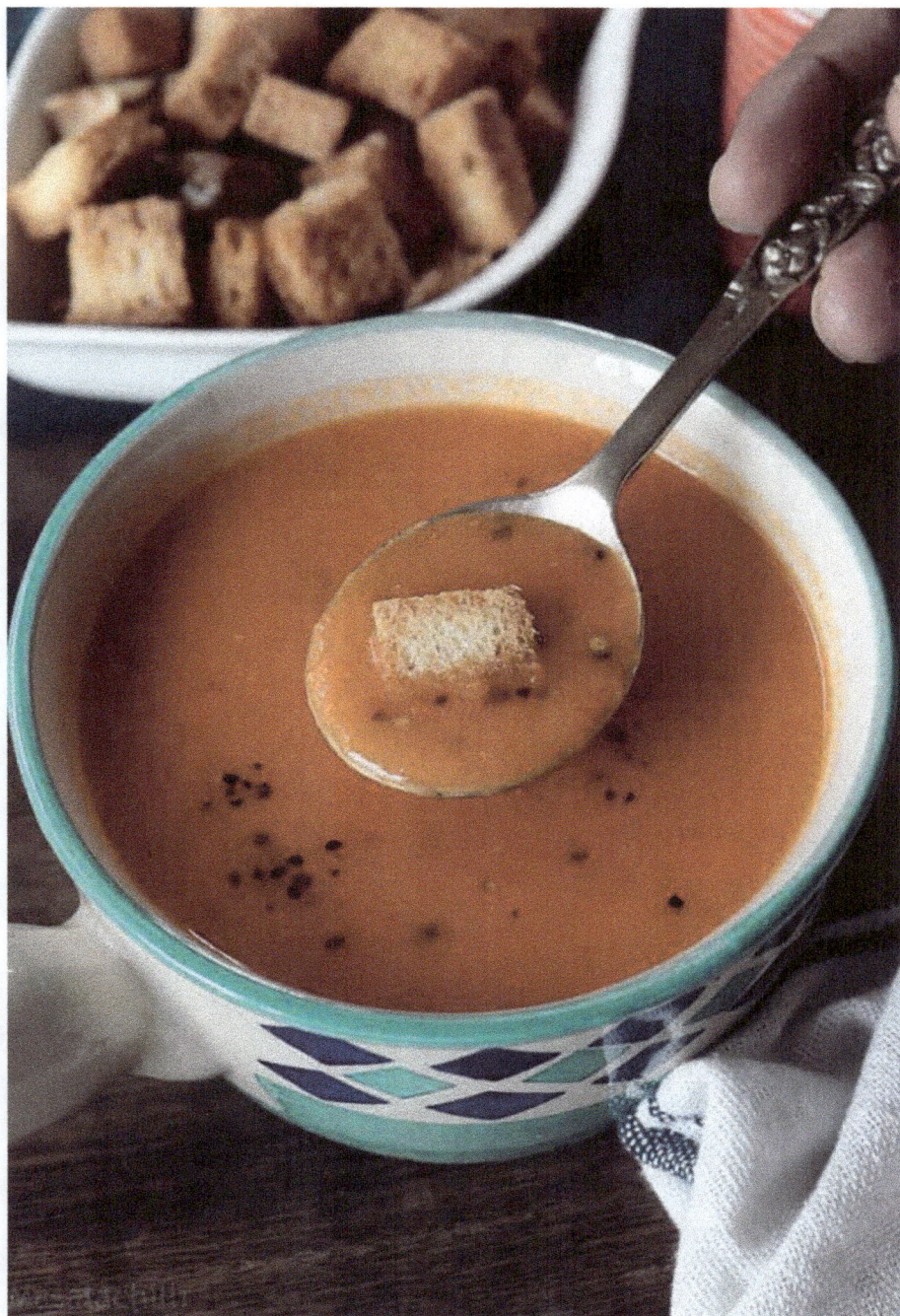

Chickpeas Soup

Prep Time: 10 min

Cook Time: 35 min

Serve: 4

Ingredients:

- 1 bunch kale, leaves torn
- Salt and black pepper to taste
- 3 tbsp. olive oil
- 1 celery stalk, chopped
- 1 yellow onion, chopped
- 1 carrot, chopped
- 30 oz. canned chickpeas, drained
- 14 oz. canned tomatoes, chopped
- 1 bay leaf
- 3 rosemary sprigs
- 4 cups veggie stock

Preparation:

1. In a bowl, mix kale with half of the oil, salt and pepper, toss to coat., spread on a lined baking sheet, cook at 425°F for 12 minutes and leave aside to cool down.

2. Heat a saucepan with remaining oil over medium high heat, add carrot, celery, onion, salt and pepper, and stir and cook for 5 minutes. Add the rest of the ingredients, toss and simmer for 20 minutes.

3. Discard rosemary and bay leaf, puree using a blender and divide into soup bowls. Top with roasted kale and serve.

Fish Soup

Prep Time: 10 min

Cook Time: 35 min

Serve: 6

Ingredients:

- 2 garlic cloves, minced

- 2 tbsp. olive oil

- 1 fennel bulb, sliced

- 1 yellow onion, chopped

- 1 pinch saffron, soaked in some orange juice for 10 minutes and drained

- 14 oz. canned tomatoes, peeled

- 1 strip orange zest

- 6 cups seafood stock

- 10 halibut fillet, cut into big pieces

- 20 shrimp, peeled and deveined

- 1 bunch parsley, chopped

- Salt and white pepper to taste

Preparation:

1. 2. Heat a saucepan with oil over medium high heat, add onion, garlic and fennel, stir and cook for 10 minutes.
Add saffron, tomatoes, orange zest and stock, stir, bring to a boil and simmer for 20 minutes.
3. Add fish and shrimp, stir and cook for 6 minutes.
4. Sprinkle parsley, salt and pepper, divide into bowls and serve.

Chili Watermelon Soup

Prep Time: 4 h

Cook Time: 5 min

Serve: 4

Ingredients:

- 3 lb. watermelon, sliced

- ½ tsp. chipotle chili powder

- 2 tbsp. olive oil

- Salt to taste

- 1 tomato, chopped

- 1 tbsp. shallot, chopped

- ¼ cup cilantro, chopped

- 1 small cucumber, chopped

- 1 small Serrano chili pepper, chopped

- 3 and ½ tbsp. lime juice

- ¼ cup crème Fraiche

- ½ tbsp. red wine vinegar

Preparation:

1. In a bowl, mix 1 tbsp. oil with chipotle powder, stir and brush the watermelon with this mix. Put the watermelon slices preheated grill pan over medium high heat, grill for 1 minute on each side, cool down, chop and put in a blender.
2. Add cucumber and the rest of the ingredients except the vinegar and the lime juice and pulse well.
3. Transfer to bowls, top with lime juice and vinegar, keep in the fridge for 4 hours and then serve.

Shrimp Soup

Prep Time: 30 min

Cook Time: 5 min

Serve: 6

Ingredients:

- 1 English cucumber, chopped
- 3 cups tomato juice
- 3 jarred roasted red peppers, chopped
- ½ cup olive oil
- 2 tbsp. sherry vinegar
- 1 tsp. sherry vinegar
- garlic clove, mashed
- baguette slices, cut into cubes and toasted
- Salt and black pepper to taste
- ½ tsp. cumin, ground

- ¾ lb. shrimp, peeled and deveined

- 1 tsp. thyme, chopped

Preparation:

1. In a blender, mix cucumber with tomato juice, red peppers and pulse well, bread, 6 tbsp. oil, 2 tbsp. vinegar, cumin, salt, pepper and garlic, pulse again, transfer to a bowl and keep in the fridge for 30 minutes.

2. Heat a saucepan with 1 tbsp. oil over high heat, add shrimp, stir and cook for 2 minutes. Add thyme, and the rest of the ingredients, cook for 1 minute and transfer to a plate.

3. Divide cold soup into bowls, top with shrimp and serve.

Halibut and Veggies Stew

Prep Time: 10 min

Cook Time: 50 min

Serve: 4

Ingredients:

- 1 yellow onion, chopped

- 2 tbsp. oil

- 1 fennel bulb, stalks removed, sliced and roughly chopped

- 1 carrot, thinly sliced crosswise

- 1 red bell pepper, chopped

- 2 garlic cloves, minced

- 3 tbsp. tomato paste

- 16 oz. canned chickpeas, drained

- ½ cup dry white wine

- tsp. thyme, chopped

- A pinch of smoked paprika

- Salt and black pepper to taste

- 1 bay leaf

- pinches saffron

- 4 baguette slices, toasted

- 3 and ½ cups water

- 13 mussels, debearded

- 11 oz. halibut fillets, skinless and cut into chunks

Preparation:

1. Heat a saucepan with the oil over medium high heat, add fennel, onion, bell pepper, garlic, tomato paste and carrot, stir and cook for 5 minutes.

2. Add wine, stir and cook for 2 minutes. Add the rest of the ingredients except the halibut and mussels, stir, bring to a boil, cover and boil for 25 minutes. Add, halibut and mussels, cover and simmer for 6 minutes more.

3. Discard unopened mussels, ladle into bowls and serve with toasted bread on the side.

Cucumber Soup

Prep Time: 10 min

Cook Time: 6 min

Serve: 4

Ingredients:

- 3 bread slices

- ¼ cup almonds

- 4 tsp. almonds

- 3 cucumbers, peeled and chopped

- 3 garlic cloves, minced

- ½ cup warm water

- 6 scallions, thinly sliced

- ¼ cup white wine vinegar

- 3 tbsp. olive oil

- Salt to taste

- 1 tsp. lemon juice

- ½ cup green grapes, cut in halves

Preparation:

1. Heat a pan over medium high heat, add almonds, stir, toast for 5 minutes, transfer to a plate and leave aside.

2. Soak bread in warm water for 2 minutes, transfer to a blender, add almost all the cucumber, salt, the oil, garlic, 5 scallions, lemon juice, vinegar and half of the almonds and pulse well. Ladle soup into bowls, top with reserved ingredients and 2 tbsp. grapes and serve.

Chickpeas, Tomato and Kale Stew

Prep Time: 10 min

Cook Time: 30 min

Serve: 4

Ingredients:

- 1 yellow onion, chopped

- tbsp. extra-virgin olive oil

- cups sweet potatoes, peeled and chopped

- 1 ½ tsp. cumin, ground

- 4-inch cinnamon stick

- 14 oz. canned tomatoes, chopped

- 14 oz. canned chickpeas, drained 1 ½ tsp. honey

- 6 tbsp. orange juice 1 cup water

- Salt and black pepper to taste

- ½ cup green olives, pitted

- 2 cups kale leaves, chopped

Preparation:

1. Heat a saucepan with the oil over medium high heat, add onion, cumin and cinnamon stir and cook for 5 minutes.

2. Add potatoes and the rest of the ingredients except the kale, stir, cover, reduce heat to medium-low and cook for 15 minutes. Add kale, stir, cover again and cook for 10 minutes more. Divide into bowls and serve.

Veggie Stew

Prep Time: 10 min

Cook Time: 50 min

Serve: 4

Ingredients:

- eggplants, chopped

- Salt and black pepper to taste

- 6 zucchinis, chopped

- 2 yellow onions, chopped

- 3 red bell peppers, chopped

- 56 oz. canned tomatoes, chopped

- A handful black olives, pitted and chopped

- A pinch of allspice, ground

- A pinch of cinnamon, ground

- 1 tsp. oregano, dried

- A drizzle of honey

- 1 tbsp. garbanzo bean flour mixed with

- 1 tbsp. water A drizzle of olive oil

- A pinch of red chili flakes

- 3 tbsp. Greek yogurt

Preparation:

1. Heat a saucepan with the oil over medium high heat, add bell peppers, onions, salt and pepper, and stir and sauté for 4 minutes.

2. Add eggplant and the rest of the ingredients except the flour, olives, chili flakes and the yogurt, stir, bring to a boil, cover, reduce heat to medium-low and cook for 45 minutes.

3. Add the remaining ingredients except the yogurt, stir, cook for 1 minute, divide into bowls and serve with some Greek yogurt on top.

Beef and Eggplant Soup

Prep Time: 10 min

Cook Time: 30 min

Serve: 8

Ingredients:

- 1 yellow onion, chopped

- 1 tbsp. olive oil

- 1 garlic clove, minced

- 1 lb. beef, ground

- 1 lb. eggplant, chopped

- ¾ cup celery, chopped

- ¾ cup carrots, chopped

- Salt and black pepper to taste

- 29 oz. canned tomatoes, drained and chopped

- 28 oz. beef stock

- ½ tsp. nutmeg, ground

- ½ cup macaroni

- 2 tsp. parsley, chopped

- ½ cup parmesan cheese, grated

Preparation:

1. Heat a large saucepan with the oil over medium heat, add onion, garlic and meat, stir and brown for 5 minutes.
2. Add celery, carrots and the other ingredients except the macaroni and the cheese, stir, bring to a simmer and cook for 20 minutes. Add macaroni, stir and cook for 12 minutes.
3. Ladle into soup bowls, top with grated cheese and serve.

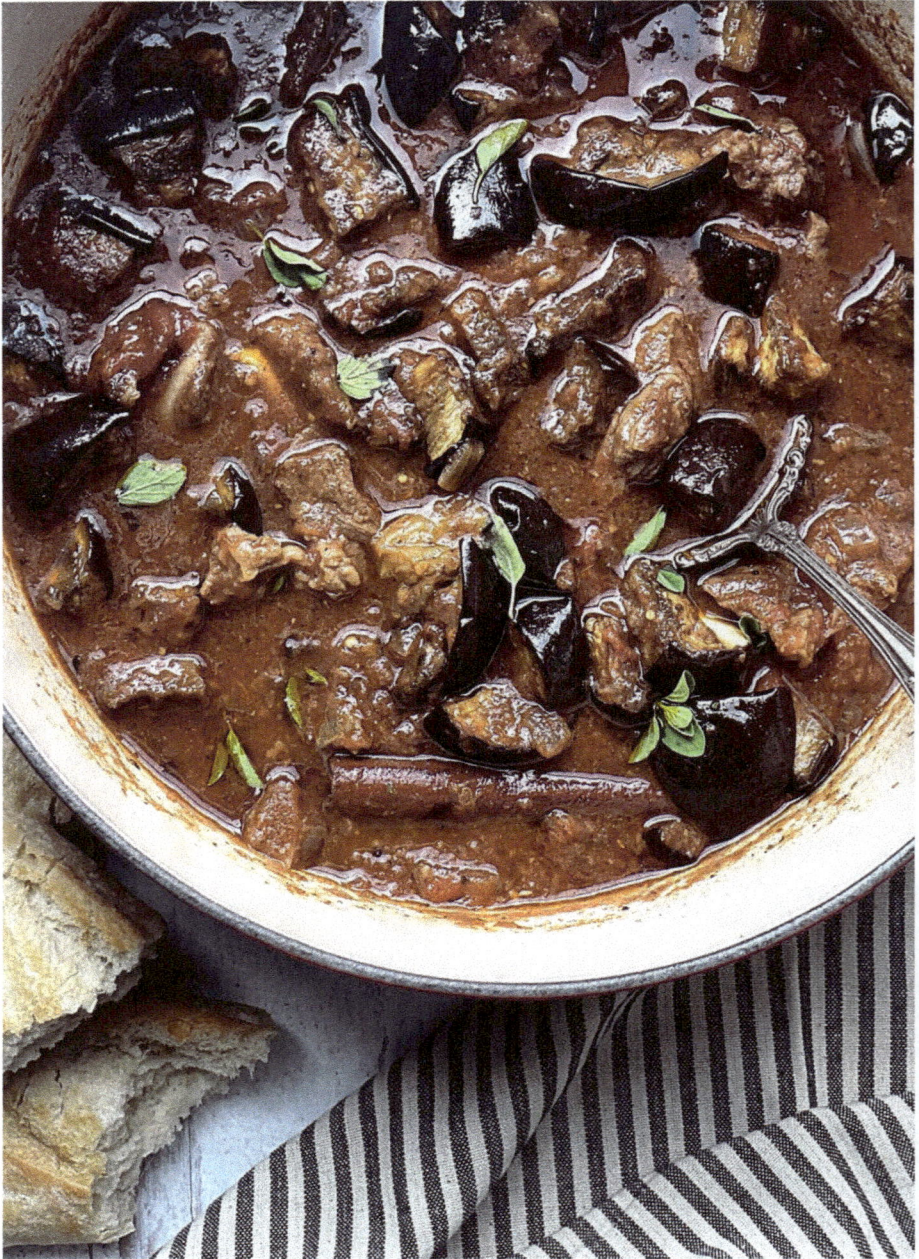

Mediterranean Greens

Preparation

Prep Time: 10 min

Cook Time: 0 min

Serve: 4

Ingredients:

- 6 cups assorted fresh mixed greens (such as radicchio, arugula, watercress, baby spinach, and romaine)
- 1 small red onion, thinly sliced
- 20 cherry tomatoes, halved
- ¼ cup dried cranberries
- ¼ cup chopped walnuts
- Crumbled feta cheese
- Freshly ground pepper to taste
- 2 tbsp. balsamic vinegar

- 2 cloves fresh garlic, finely minced

- 4 tbsp. extra-virgin olive oil

- 1 tbsp. water

- ½ tsp. crushed dried oregano

Preparation:

1. Take out a large salad bowl, combine walnuts, greens, tomatoes, onion, and cranberries. Gently toss.

2. For the dressing, combine water, vinegar, oregano, olive oil, and garlic. Mix the ingredients well. Pour over the salad and lightly toss. Add feta cheese as garnish, if preferred.

3. Add pepper to taste.

Classic Greek Salad

Prep Time: 15 min

Cook Time: 0 min

Serve: 6

Ingredients:

- 6 large firm tomatoes, quartered

- 20 Greek black olives

- ½ lb. Greek feta cheese, cut into small cubes

- ½ head of escarole, shredded

- 3 tbsp. red wine vinegar

- ¼ cup extra-virgin olive oil

- 1 tbsp. dried oregano

- ½ English cucumber, peeled, seeded, and thinly sliced

- 2 cloves fresh garlic, finely minced

- ½ red onion, sliced

- 1 medium red bell pepper, seeded and sliced

- ¼ cup freshly chopped Italian parsley

- Salt and freshly ground pepper to taste

Preparation:

1. Take out a large bowl and add vinegar, oregano, olive oil, and garlic. Add salt and pepper to taste. Set aside the bowl.

2. In another large bowl, add onion, tomatoes, escarole, cucumber, bell pepper, and cheese and mix them well.

3. Take the vinegar mixture and pour it over the salad in the second bowl. Top the salad with olives and parsley.

North African Zucchini Salad

Prep Time: 10 min

Cook Time: 0 min

Serve: 4

Ingredients:

- 1 lb. firm green zucchini, thinly sliced

- ½ tsp. ground cumin

- 2 cloves fresh garlic, finely minced

- Juice from 1 large lemon

- 1 tbsp. extra-virgin olive oil

- 1½ tbsp. plain low-fat yogurt

- Crumbled feta cheese

- Finely chopped parsley for garnish

- Salt and freshly ground pepper to taste

Preparation:

1. Add the zucchini into a large saucepan and steam it for about 2-5 minutes, or until it becomes tender and crispy. Place the zucchini under cold water and drain well.

2. Take out a large bowl and mix cumin, olive oil, lemon juice, garlic, and yogurt. Add salt and pepper to taste. Add the zucchini into the mixture in the bowl and toss gently.

3. Serve with feta cheese and parsley as garnish.

Tunisian Style Carrot Salad

Prep Time: 15 min

Cook Time: 0 min

Serve: 6

Ingredients:

- 10 medium carrots, peeled and sliced
- 1 cup crumbled feta cheese, divided
- 2 tsp. caraway seed
- ¼ cup extra-virgin olive oil
- 6 tbsp. apple cider vinegar
- 5 tsp. freshly minced garlic
- 1 tbsp. Harissa paste (choose the level of heat based on your preference)
- 20 pitted Kalamata olives, reserving some for garnish
- Salt to taste

Preparation:

1. Take out a medium saucepan and place it on medium heat. Fill it with water and add the carrots. Cook carrots until tender. Drain and cool the carrots under cold water. Drain again to remove any excess water.

2. Take out a large bowl and place the carrots in them.

3. Take out a mortar and combine salt, garlic, and caraway seeds. Grind them until they form a paste. Otherwise, you can also use a small bowl, preferably one not made out of glass for grind. The final option would be to toss the ingredients into a blender and pulse them. Add vinegar and Harissa into the bowl with the carrots and mix them well.

4. Use a large spoon and mash the carrots. Add the garlic mixture into the carrot and mix again until they have all blended well. Add the olive oil and mix again.

5. Finally, add about ½ the feta cheese and all the olives and mix well again. Take out a large bowl and add the salad to it. Top it with the remaining feta cheese.

Caesar Salad

Prep Time: 5 min

Cook Time: 0 min

Serve: 6

Ingredients:

- 10 small pitted black olives, chopped
- 1-2 bunches romaine lettuce, cleaned and torn in pieces
- 2 tsp. lemon juice
- 2½ tsp. balsamic vinegar
- ½ cup grated parmesan cheese
- ½ cup nonfat plain yogurt
- 1 tsp. worcestershire sauce
- ½ tsp. anchovy paste
- 2 cloves freshly minced garlic

Preparation:

1. Take out a large bowl and place romaine lettuce in it.

2. Take out your blended and add mix lemon juice, yogurt, garlic, anchovy paste, vinegar, worcestershire sauce, and ¼ cup parmesan cheese. Mix all the ingredients well until they are smooth.

3. Pour the yogurt mixture over the lettuce and toss lightly.

4. Top the salad with the remaining parmesan cheese.

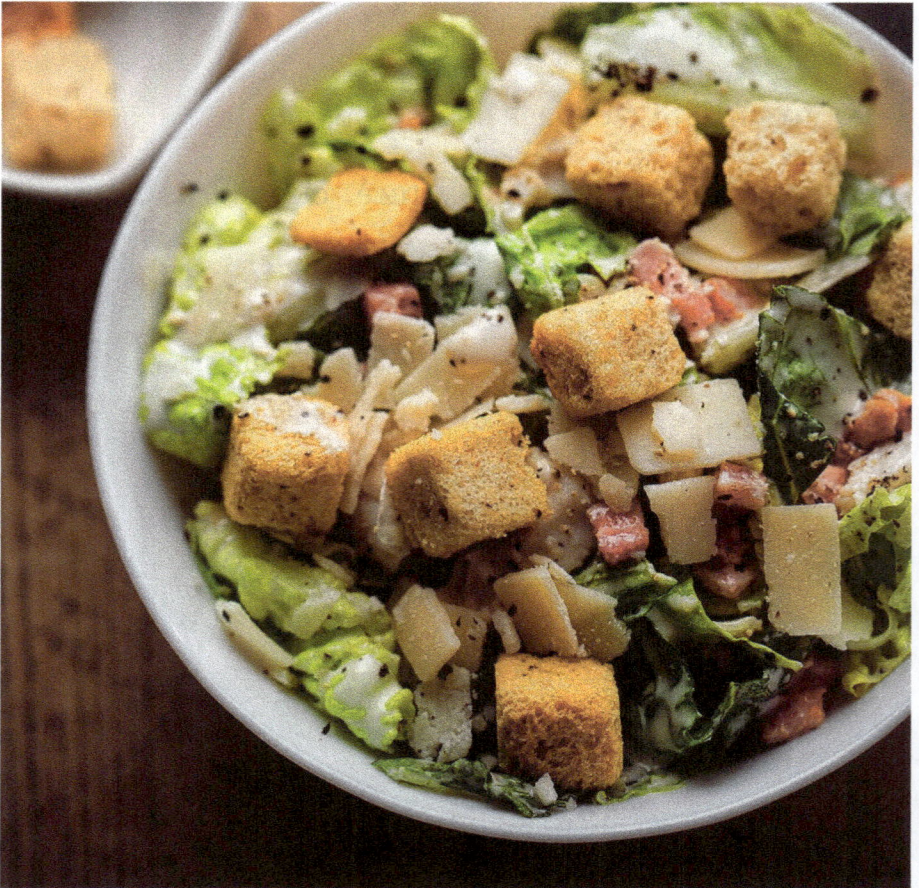

Cress and Tangerine Salad

Prep Time: 15 min

Cook Time: 0 min

Serve: 4

Ingredients:

- 4 large sweet tangerines

- ¼ cup extra-virgin olive oil

- 2 large bunches watercress, washed and stems removed Juice from 1 fresh lemon

- 10 cherry tomatoes, halved

- 16 pitted Kalamata olives

- Sea salt and freshly ground pepper to taste

Preparation:

1. Take the tangerines and peel them into a medium-sized bowl. Make sure that you remove any pits and squeeze the sections. You should have around ¼ cup of tangerine juice.

Set sections aside. Take a large bowl and add lemon juice, tangerine juice, and olive oil. Mix them and add salt and pepper for flavor, if you prefer.

2. Use paper towels to pat the cress dry. Add watercress, tomatoes, and olives to the bowl containing the tangerine sections (not to be confused with the bowl containing tangerine juice). Toss them lightly.

3. Pour the tangerine juice mixture on top. Mix well and serve.

Prosciutto and Figs Salad

Prep Time: 10 min

Cook Time: 0 min

Serve: 4

Ingredients:

- One 10-12-oz. package fresh baby spinach

- 1 small hot red chili pepper, finely diced

- 1 carton figs, stems removed and quartered

- ½ cup walnuts, coarsely chopped

- 1 tbsp. fresh orange juice

- 1 tbsp. honey

- 4 slices prosciutto, cut into strips

- Shaved parmesan cheese for garnish

Preparation:

1. Take your spinach and divide them into 4 equal portions. Each portion should be on a separate plate and will act as a base. Add quartered prosciutto, figs, and walnuts on each spinach as toppings.

2. For the dressing, take a small bowl and add honey, orange juice, and diced pepper. Add the mixture over the salad.

3. Finally, toss the salad lightly and use parmesan cheese for the garnish.

Garden Vegetables and Chickpeas Salad

Prep Time: 10 min

Cook Time: 0 min

Serve: 4

Ingredients:

- 2 tbsp. freshly squeezed lemon juice

- 1/8 tsp. freshly ground pepper

- 1 cup cubed part-skim mozzarella cheese

- 1 tbsp. fresh basil leaf, snipped

- 1 (15-oz.) can chickpeas, rinsed and well drained

- 2 cups coarsely chopped fresh broccoli

- 2 cloves fresh garlic, finely minced

- ½ cup sliced fresh carrots

- 1 7½-oz. can diced tomatoes, undrained

Preparation:

1. Use a large bowl and add garlic, basil, lemon juice, and ground pepper. Mix them well.

2. Add the chickpeas, carrots, tomatoes with juice, broccoli, and mozzarella cheese. Toos all the ingredients well.

3. You can serve immediately, or you can keep it refrigerated overnight.

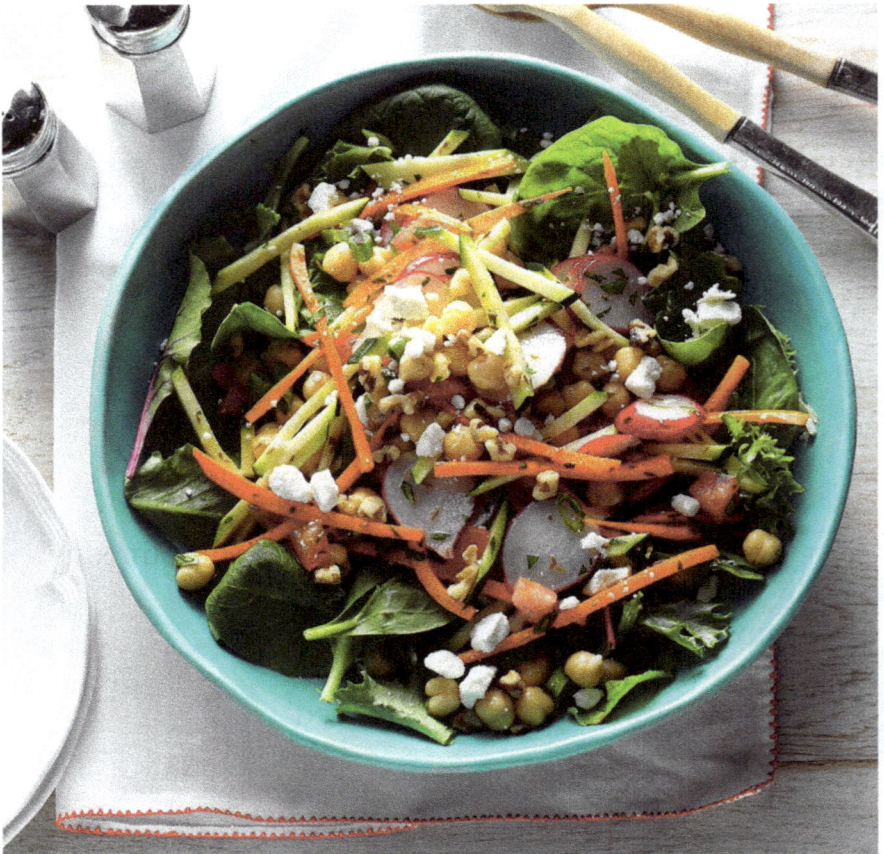

Peppered Watercress Salad

Prep Time: 5 min

Cook Time: 0 min

Serve: 4

Ingredients:

- 2 tsp. champagne vinegar
- 2 bunches (about 8 cups) watercress, rinsed and rough stems removed
- 2 tbsp. extra-virgin olive oil
- Salt and freshly ground pepper to taste

Preparation:

1. Drain the watercress properly.

2. Take out a small bowl and then add salt, pepper, vinegar, and olive oil. Mix them well together. Transfer the watercress to a bowl. Add the vinegar mixture into it and toss well. Serve immediately.

Baked egg with cheddar and beef

Prep Time: 20 min

Cook Time: 20 min

Serve: 6

Ingredients:

- Six eggs 1 lb beef
- One chopped green pepper
- Salt to taste
- Pepper to taste
- 1 cup green beans
- Cream of mushroom soup
- 1/2 cup shredded cheddar cheese
- 1 cup almond milk
- 1 tbsp vegetable oil
- 1 cup mushrooms

- 1 tsp onion powder

- 2 tbsp cornstarch

- 1/2 tsp salt

Preparation:

1. Cook beef with beans and bell pepper. Crack eggs and cook for five minutes.

2. Transfer the beef to the casserole and pour mushroom soup and toss. Bake in a preheated oven at 350 degrees for 20 minutes.

Cream of Mushroom Soup:

1. Blend all the items of mushroom soup in the blender.

2. Boil the mixture and simmer it for 12 minutes.

Heavenly egg bake with pancakes

Prep Time: 15 min

Cook Time: 25 min

Serve: 8

Ingredients:

- 2 cups baking mix
- 2 cups shredded Cheddar cheese
- 1 cup milk
- 5 tbsp maple syrup
- Two eggs
- 1.5 tbsp white sugar
- 12 slices cooked bacon

Preparation:

1. Mix all the ingredients in a bowl and bake in a preheated oven at 350 degrees for 25 minutes.

2. Top with cheese and bacon and bake for five more minutes.

Blueberry and vanilla scones

Prep Time: 15 min

Cook Time: 10 min

Serve: 8

Ingredients:

- 1/2 tsp baking powder

- 225 g Self-rising flour

- One pinch of salt

- 2 tbsp soured cream

- One egg

- 50 g caster sugar

- 75 g butter

- 75 g blueberries

- 1 tsp vanilla extract

Preparation:

1. Mix flour, salt, baking powder, sugar, butter, and blueberries in a bowl.

2. Whisk vanilla with cream and egg and add in flour mixture. Make small rounded shapes and bake in a preheated oven at 200 degrees for 15 minutes.

3. Mix strawberries, sugar, and vanilla and make syrup.

4. Pour syrup over baked cookies and serve.

Frittata with brie and bacon

Prep Time: 5 min

Cook Time: 20 min

Serve: 6

Ingredients:

- 1/2 tsp salt

- 1/2 tsp pepper

- 1/2 cup whipping cream

- Eight slices bacon

- Eight eggs

- Two cloves garlic

- 4 oz brie

Preparation:

1. Heat oil in a skillet over medium flame and saute bacon for five minutes. Transfer bacon to plate.

2. Mix egg, cream salt, bacon, pepper, and garlic and cook in heated oil over medium flame. Broil bacon mixture for five minutes in broiler over a high flame.

Coffee with butter

Prep Time: 5 min

Cook Time: 5 min

Serve: 1

Ingredients:

- 1 cup hot coffee

- 2 tbsp butter

- 1 tbsp coconut oil

Preparation:

Combine all the items in a blender and serve.

Pecorino pasta with sausage and tomato

Prep Time: 20 min

Cook Time: 20 min

Serve: 4

Ingredients:

- 2 tsp olive oil
- 1 cup sliced onion
- 8 oz penne
- 8 oz Italian sausage
- 6 tbsp grated Romano cheese
- 1/4 tsp salt
- 2 tsp garlic
- 1 1/4 lb tomatoes
- 1/8 tsp black pepper
- 1/4 cup torn basil leaves

Preparation:

1. Boil & drain pasta. Keep the boiled pasta aside.

2. Now at a full flame, heat a skillet, which should be nonstick. Take oil in a pan & add sausage and onion to it.

3. Cook for about two minutes. Now remove from stove & add pasta, salt, black pepper powder & cheese. Add oil to a pan, swirl to coat. Sprinkle remaining 1/4th cup of cheese and serve.

Pesto pasta and shrimp

Prep Time: 10 min

Cook Time: 10 min

Serve: 3

Ingredients:

- 10 oz spaghetti

- 3/4 cup basil pesto

- 1 lb shrimp

- 1 tbsp olive oil

- 1 tsp Italian seasoning

- Salt to taste

- Black pepper to taste

- 1/4 cup parmesan cheese

Preparation:

1. Bring a pot of salted water to a boil and cook the pasta. While the pasta is cooking, prepare the shrimp. Heat the olive oil in a pan over high heat.

2. Add the shrimp and sprinkle with Italian seasoning, salt, and pepper. Cook for 2-4 minutes or until shrimp is just pink and opaque. Turn off the heat.

3. Drain the pasta and add it to the pan with the shrimp. Stir in the pesto. Add the cherry tomatoes and parmesan cheese to the pan. Garnish with parsley if desired.

Spanish rice casserole with cheesy beef

Prep Time: 10 min

Cook Time: 25 min

Serve: 4

Ingredients:

- 16.8 oz Spanish Rice mix

- 1 tbsp olive oil

- One red bell pepper

- 1 cup of corn

- 1 cup meatless crumbles

- 1/3 cup sour cream

- 1/4 cup salsa

- 1/2 cup Monterey Jack cheese

- 2 tbsp crumbled queso fresco

- One avocado sliced

Preparation:

1. Prepare the rice in a 2.5-liter casserole dish, which should be microwavable. Preheat the microwave up to 375 F.

2. Take a skillet and heat the oil. Now cook bell pepper till tendered 5-7 minutes. Once the rice is cooked, then combine the bell pepper, cooked, meatless crumbles, salsa, sour cream & corn. Now sprinkle the cheese on the top.

3. Bake it, uncovered (10 minutes), till the cheese is melted & browned on top. Top sliced avocado.

Yangchow Chinese style fried rice

Prep Time: 15 min

Cook Time: 20 min

Serve: 6

Ingredients:

- 6 cups cooked white rice
- 1 cup barbecued pork
- 1 tsp sugars
- 1 tsp ginger
- Ten pieces of shrimps
- 3/4 cup green peas
- 1 tsp garlic
- 1 1/2 tbsp soy sauce
- 2 tsp salt
- 1/4 cup green onion

- Two beaten eggs

- 3 tbsp cooking oil

Preparation:

1. Heat the oil & sauté ginger-garlic together. Add the shrimps & cook (1 minute). Pour the egg mixture & cook.

2. Divide the cooked egg into pieces. Add rice & soy sauce, salt & sugar, and mix with other ingredients.

3. Add pork, which is barbecued & cook (3 minutes). Add peas & shrimp & cook 3 minutes. Add onions and cook (2 minutes). Turn off heat & transfer to a serving plate.

Mahi-mahi pomegranate sauce

Prep Time: 5 min

Cook Time: 20 min

Serve: 2

Ingredients:

- 12 oz Mahi-mahi fillets

- 1/2 cup balsamic vinegar

- 1/4 cup pomegranate juice

- 1 tbsp olive oil

- 1 tbsp squeezed lemon juice

- 1/2 cup pomegranate seeds

Preparation:

1. Preheat microwave up to 450 deg. Take baking dish & lay

Mahi fillets, drizzle with lemon juice & olive oil.

2. Bake it for 15-20 minutes Take a pan & heat vinegar, pomegranate juice & seeds over high heat.

3. Bring a boil & let the sauce to reduce (20 minutes). Spoon the fillets. Serve & enjoy.

Feta tomato sea bass

Prep Time: 10 min

Cook Time: 10 min

Serve: 4

Ingredients:

- 2 oz dry white wine

- 2 tbsp lemon juice

- 32 oz sea bass fillets

- 4 oz feta cheese

- Five ripe tomatoes

- 5 tbsp olive oil

- 2 tbsp butter

- 2 tbsp basil

- Three garlic cloves

- 1 tbsp oregano

- Salt & pepper

Preparation:

1. Take fish & rub salt & pepper over it. Heat the pan & add olive oil. Put the fish in a pan.

2. Cook it until it is golden brown. Add basil, cheese, lemon juice, tomatoes & garlic. Bake 12-15 minutes at 400 deg. Take the dish out and finish it with butter.

3. The dish is ready. Now serve and enjoy.

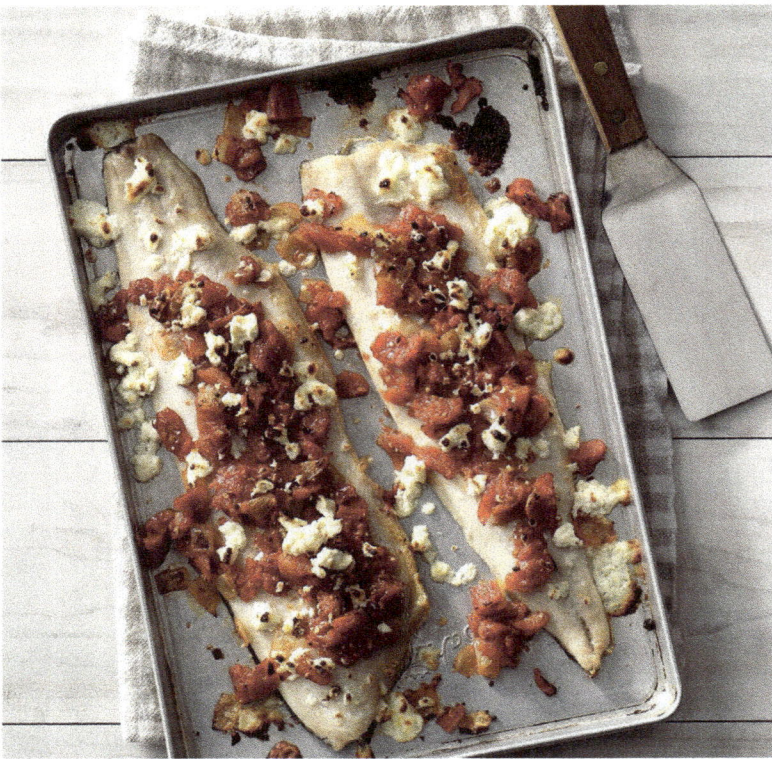

Crab stew

Prep Time: 25 min

Cook Time: 25 min

Serve: 4

Ingredients:

- 2 tbsp sweet paprika

- 1/2 cup heavy cream

- 6 tbsp unsalted butter

- 1/4 lb shrimp

- 1 lb lump crabmeat

- 2 cups steamed rice

- 3/4 tsp chipotle Chile powder

- 2 tbsp all-purpose flour

- 1/4 cup dry sherry

- 2 cups clam juice

- 1 cup of water

- One small onion

- One garlic clove

- Salt and pepper

- 1 tbsp leaf parsley

Preparation:

1. Melt one tbsp of butter in a pan. Add shrimp & cook at moderate heat. Now add sherry & cook for 2 minutes.

2. Add clam juice & water. Bring a boil & simmer moderately at low heat for 10 minutes. Strain broth. Now again, melt 2 tbsp butter in the pan. Add garlic & onion & cook at moderate heat till it is softened. Add paprika & chipotle, stirring for 3 minutes. Now stir with flour. Whisk broth in the pan. Cook till it becomes smooth & then bring a boil. Simmer at low heat. Whisk till it is just thickened 5 minutes. Add cream, simmer & season with salt & pepper.

3. Take a skillet & melt 3 tbsp butter. Now gently stir the crab & cook at moderate heat. Toss for a few minutes' till warmed 4 minutes. Season with salt & pepper, Spoon steamed rice into the shallow bowls, Ladle shellfish sauce on rice & top with crab. Sprinkle with parsley & serve.

Savory zucchini loaf

Prep Time: 25 min

Cook time: 50-55 min

Serve: 8

Ingredients:

- 5 tbsp of olive oil

- One small, diced zucchini.

- Half cup of hazelnuts.

- ¾ cup of tomato (sun-dried).

- Half cup milk

- One cup all-purpose flour

- Three eggs

- 2 tsp of baking powder

- 2/3 cup of mozzarella cheese.

- ¼ cup of basil.

- ¼ tbsp of black pepper

- ¼ tbsp of sea salt

Preparation:

1. Preheat the microwave up to 350 F Toast hazelnuts on moderate heat in a frypan. Sauté diced zucchini on medium heat (5 min). Place tomatoes in a bowl. For ten minutes, cover it with hot water. Drain it and place it aside.

2. Take three eggs and whisk them in a bowl. Add milk to eggs & beat. Add flour & baking soda mix until it becomes smooth. Add 5 tbsp of olive oil & pepper. Mix it well.

3. Add other ingredients tomatoes, basil, hazelnuts & mozzarella. Mix delicately with a spatula. Spray the pan with cooking spray & pour the batter into it. Bake for almost 45 min until toothpick comes out dry and clean. Cut it into slices & serve.

Chilled Pea and mint soup

Prep Time: 20 min

Cook Time: 20-25 min

Serve: 4

Ingredients:

- 2 tbsp of butter

- One chopped onion medium size.

- Two cups of water

- Two pounds of frozen green peas

- Two cups of vegetable broth.

- ¼ cup of fresh mint leaves

- ¼ cup of fresh parsley

- 1 tsp of fresh lemon juice

- Half tsp cayenne

- Mint leaves for garnishing

Preparation:

1. Melt the butter in a large pan. Add onions & cook till softened for 7 minutes. Combine vegetable stock & water in a medium-sized saucepan.

2. Stir in 1/2 of the water mixture in the large pan along with the onions. Increase the heat & bring to boil. Add peas & bring to a boil for one minute. Remove from stove.

3. Add remaining water mixture with the mint, parsley & cayenne. Puree with an immersion blender in a pot till it becomes smooth. Season using lime juice.

4. Cool until chilled. Serve in the bowls with mint leaves.

Watermelon & cantaloupe salad

Prep Time: 10 min

Cook Time: 0 min

Serve: 6

Ingredients:

- ¼ cup of pine nuts

- 2 cups of diced cantaloupe

- Six cups of diced watermelon

- 5 tbsp of olive oil

- 2/3 cup of crumbled feta cheese

- 1/4 cup of fresh mint.

- ¼ tsp of black pepper powder

Preparation:

1. Toast pine nuts in a pan. Add olive oil, cantaloupe & watermelon in a bowl. Sprinkle the cheese, mint & pepper.

2. Mix it delicately. Chill for one hour. Serve.

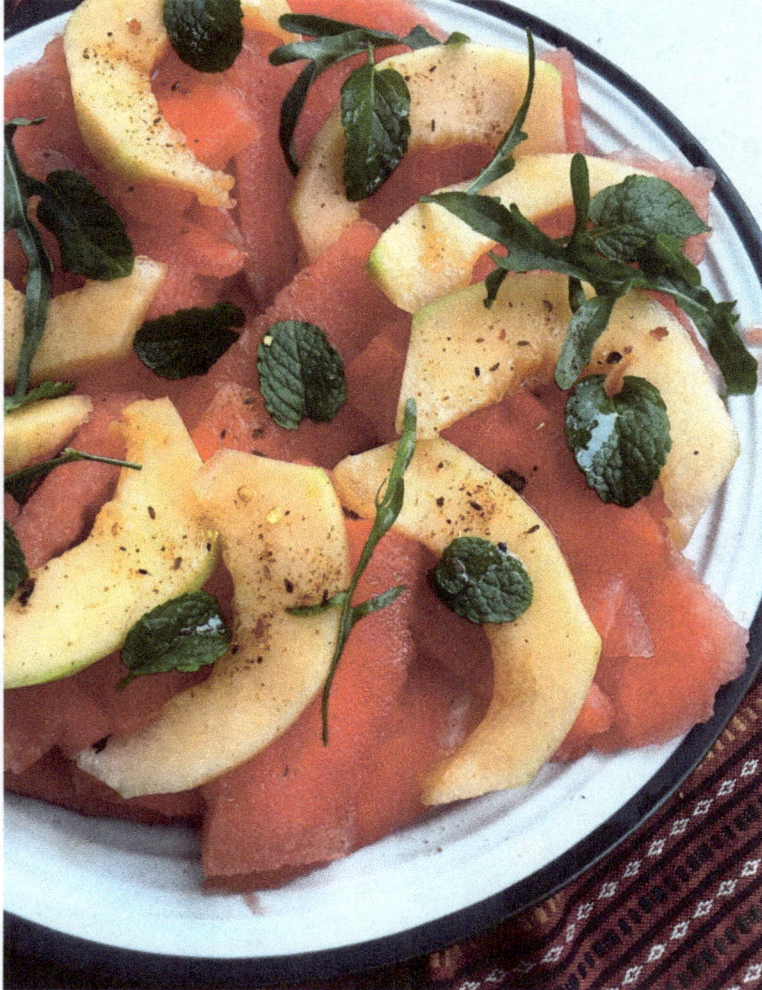

Southern-fried okra

Prep Time: 5 min

Cook Time: 25 min

Serve: 6

Ingredients:

- Half cup flour-unbleached

- Half cup of cornmeal.

- 1/8th tsp of salt

- 1/4th tsp of fresh black pepper

- One egg

- Two tbsp of milk

- 1/3rd cup of sunflower oil

- 3 cups of fresh okra

Preparation:

1. Preheat the microwave up to 300 F. Mix & whisk together the flour, salt, black pepper & cayenne in a bowl.

2. Beat egg & milk in a bowl. Heat sunflower oil.

3. Dip okra pieces in the egg batter & roll in a mixture.

4. Fry in the pan. Turn over after two min. Remove the cooked okra with a spoon & drain each batch. Transfer 1st batch to a baking dish to keep it warm while the remaining okra is cooking.

5. Place the 2nd batch of the fried okra in the oven till the final batch is done. Serve it immediately.

Pesto Pasta with Peas and Mozzarella

Prep Time: 10 min

Cook Time: 0 min

Serve: 3

Ingredients:

- 2 cups green peas

- 1 cup mozzarella balls low sodium

- 4 cups Boiled Penna Pasta

- 2 cups fresh basil leaves

- ¼ tsp Garlic powder

- 1 tbsp Lemon juice

- 2 tsp zest of a lemon

- 1/3 cup olive oil

- ¼ tsp Salt

- ¼ tsp Pepper

Preparation:

1. For making pesto, add all the ingredients in a blender or food processor and mix them except for olive oil. Pulse until crudely sliced. Reduce the food processor's speed or blender, slowly add olive oil to it, mix it well, and blend.

2. Scrape down the sides of the food processor/blender to fully mix the end. Add salt & pepper.

3. Add mozzarella, pasta, and peas into a large bowl. Add pesto according to requirement Add pesto as desired and then mix all ingredients.

Balsamic Roasted Green Beans

Prep Time: 5 min

Cook Time: 17 min

Serve: 1 cup

Ingredients:

- 1 lb Green beans
- 2 Chopped Garlic Cloves
- 1 tbsp Balsamic vinegar
- 1 tbsp Olive oil
- ⅛ tsp Salt
- ⅛ tsp Pepper

Preparation:

1. Preheat oven to 425°F. Mix green beans along with olive oils, pepper & salt in a large bowl.

2. Evenly spread green beans on a foil or parchment paper-lined on a baking sheet. Bake them for 10-12 mints in the oven until it turns light brown.

3. Spread garlic with green beans & mix well to combine. Then again, bake it for another 5 minutes till beans are warm & browned.

4. Remove from oven & toss with balsamic vinegar.

Mac in a Flash (Macaroni and Cheese)

Prep Time: 2 min

Cook Time: 10 min

Serve: 4

Ingredients:

- 3 cups Water
- 1 cup Noodles
- ½ cup Grated Cheddar Cheese
- 1 tsp Butter
- ⅛ tsp dry mustard

Preparation:

1. Add noodles in boiling water, boil it for 5 to 7 minutes or until tender, and then drain the boiled noodles.

2. Sprinkle the grated cheddar cheese on the hot noodles & mix it with butter and dry grounded mustard.

Costa Rican Gallo Pinto

Prep Time: 5 min

Cook Time: 30 min

Serve: 4

Ingredients:

- 1/3 cup dry black beans

- 4 tbsp Olive oil

- 110g Chopped Onion

- 2 Chopped Garlic Cloves

- One chopped red bell pepper

- 1 tsp Cumin

- 1 tbsp Salsa Lizano

- 3 cups Cooked White rice

- ½ tsp black pepper

- Bit of smoked paprika

- ¼ cup Chopped Cilantro

- 4 Hard-boiled eggs

- Salt to taste

Preparation:

Preparation of beans advance:

1. Soak black beans in one and a half cups of water at least for 2 hrs. or overnight.

2. Add beans in boiling water and boil them until beans tender for ten- fifteen. Save beans along with water.

Preparation for Gallo pinto:

1. Take a large frying pan and heat the oil over medium heat.

2. Then add sliced veggies (garlic, onion, & red pepper) to it.

3. Fry and stir it while frying unless or until vegies becomes soft & aromatic. After adding cumin and salsa Lozano in it, mix, then gin cook gin for two to three more minutes.

4. Now mix the boiled bens and its water in it and again cook for just one mint. Combine the cooked rice & make sure that stir until rice is completely mixed with the beans.

5. Cover the frying pan, reduce the heat & cook again for one to two minutes, till the rice is warmed. Flavor with smoked paprika, pepper & cilantro for good flavor.

6. Finally, add this to a bowl and decorate it with a hard-boiled egg on top.

Cheese Quiche

Prep Time: 5 min

Cook Time: 45 min

Serve: 8

Ingredients:

- 4 Marginally beaten eggs
- Splash of Pepper
- 1.5 cup milk
- 3 oz shredded cheddar cheese
- ¼ cup Chopped onion
- 1 tsp Parsley leaves
- Pastry shell un-baked

Preparation:

1. Preheatooven to 350°F. Mix all ingredients in a large bowl & mix it perfectly.

2. Now add already prepared unbaked pastry shell. Bake this for forty to forty-five minutes.

3. Cut into eight slices but cool this before baking.

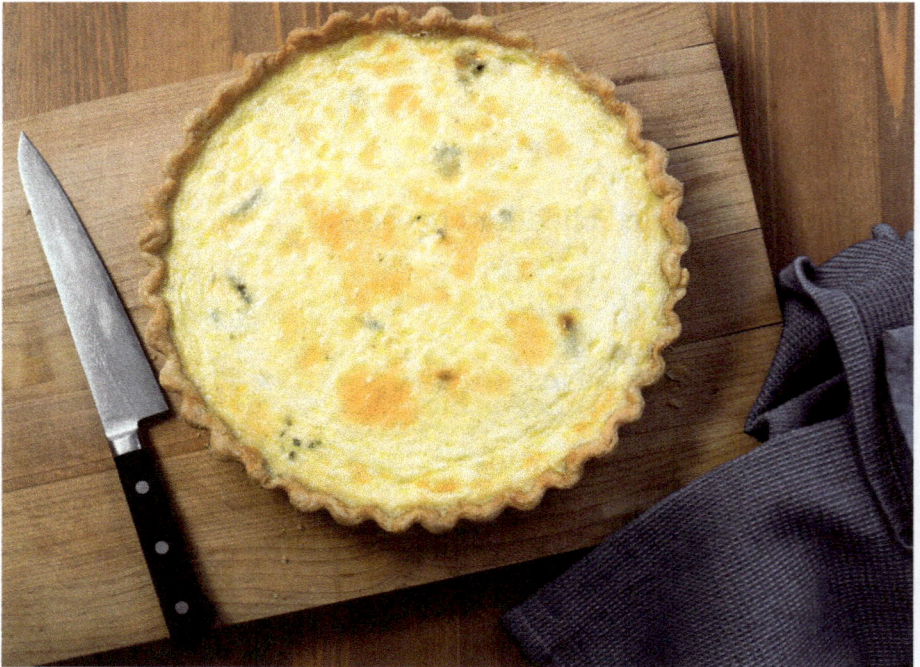

Cheesy thyme waffles

Prep Time: 10 min

Cook Time: 7 min

Serve: 2

Ingredients:

- Two eggs

- 1/3 cup parmesan cheese

- 1 tsp garlic powder

- 1 tsp thyme

- 1 cup collard greens

- 1 tbsp olive oil

- Two stalks onion

- 1/2 cauliflower

- 1/2 tsp salt

- 1 cup shredded mozzarella cheese

- 1 tbsp of sesame seeds

- 1/2 tsp black pepper

Preparation:

1. Cut cauliflower & slice onions. Add cauliflower to the blender. Add onions, thyme & collard greens to the blender & pulse again. Now add the processed mixture to a bowl.

2. Mix it well to form a smooth batter. A heat waffle iron.

3. Pour the mixture into the waffle iron, ensuring that it is spread properly. Cook well & serve hot.

Baked egg and asparagus with cheese parmesan

Prep Time: 10 min

Cook Time: 15 min

Serve: 3

Ingredients:

- 30 spears asparagus

- Six eggs

- 3 tbsp parmesan cheese

- 3/4 tsp salt

- 3 tsp butter

- 3 tsp olive oil

- 3/4 tsp black pepper

Preparation:

1. Preheat microwave up to 400 deg. Take a small pot of water. Add salt & add asparagus. Stir it well.

2. When water boils again, please remove it from the stove.

3. Drain asparagus & transfer it to a bowl filled with cold water. Distribute asparagus.

4. Among three baking dishes, Top center of the baking dish along with one tsp of butter. Season with salt.

5. Add eggs to the baking dish. Bake for 10 min. Remove it from the microwave. Top each portion with cheese & black pepper. Return to microwave & bake it for 7 min.

6. Serve and enjoy.

Creamy cold salad

Prep Time: 10 min

Cook Time: 1 min

Serve: 3

Ingredients:

- 8 oz salad macaroni
- 1/4 sliced green onion
- 1/2 cup red pepper
- 1/2 cup black olives
- 1 cup broccoli florets
- 1/2 cup cucumber

Dressing:

- 1/2 cup mayonnaise
- 2 tsp vinegar
- 1/2 tsp kosher salt

- 1/2 tsp black pepper

- 1/2 tsp sugar

Preparation:

1. Cook pasta. When noodles are cooked, add broccoli.

2. Let broccoli boil 40 sec. Drain everything. Rinse well

3. Stir with mayonnaise, salt, pepper, vinegar & sugar in a

bowl. Add cooked pasta & broccoli in a bowl & stir well.

4. Add cucumber, olives, pepper, & onion. Stir again.

5. Cover & refrigerate until the ready dish is ready to serve.

6. Stir again before serving. Enjoy the food!

Peppy pepper tomato salad

Prep Time: 5 min

Cook Time: 10 min

Serve: 4

Ingredients:

- One small garlic

- 1/4 cup olive oil

- 1 tbsp sherry vinegar

- 1 tsp balsamic vinegar

- Salt and pepper

- 1 pound tomatoes

- 1.5 pounds red peppers

- 1 tbsp basil

- One leaf lettuce

Preparation:

1. Mix sherry vinegar, garlic, olive oil, balsamic vinegar, salt, and black pepper powder according to taste. Cut roasted peppers strips. Toss with dressing.

2. Add 1/2 basil & toss again. Remove & discard tough outer leaves. Wash & dry the leaves & tear them to pieces.

3. Toss with tomatoes & dressing & basil. Line platter. Top with peppers. Serve slightly chilled.

Spinach and grilled feta salad

Prep Time: 10 min

Cook Time: 20 min

Serve: 1

Ingredients:

- 1/2 tbsp olive oil

- 1 oz feta cheese

- 1 cup shredded mozzarella cheese

- One pinch of salt

- pepper to taste

- One clove garlic

- Two ciabatta rolls

- 1/4 lb spinach

Preparation:

1. Mince garlic & add to a pan with olive oil. Cook at moderate heat for 3 minutes. Add frozen spinach & turn heat up. Cook 5 minutes. Season it lightly with sea salt & black pepper. Cut rolls in half.

2. Add shredded mozzarella & half oz. of feta to bottom. Divide cooked spinach. Then top each sandwich with a pinch of red pepper plus more mozzarella. Place top of ciabatta roll on sandwiches & transfer in a non- stick pan

3. Fill the pot with water for creating weight. Place pot on the top of sandwiches to press them. Flip sandwiches carefully. Place the weighted pot on top & cook. Serve hot and enjoy.

Salmon and Cucumber Salad

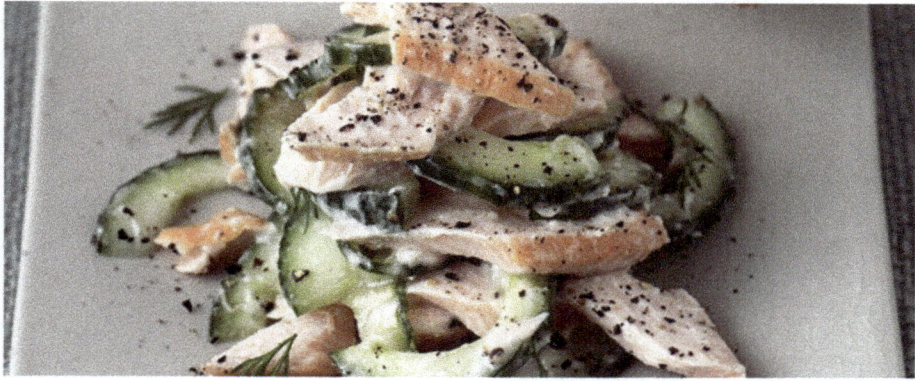

Prep Time: 8 min

Cook Time: 35 min

Serve: 4

Ingredients:

- Sauce

- 1/4 tsp kosher salt

- 2 tsp lemon juice

- 13 tsp pepper

- 1 tbsp olive oil

- 1 tbsp chopped dill

- 1 cup yogurt

- Cucumber salad

- 2 tsp olive oil

- 2 tsp chopped flat-leaf parsley

- 2 tsp chopped chives

- 13 tsp pepper

- 13 tsp kosher salt

- 1.5 tsp minced shallot

- ¾ tsp lemon juice

- ½ lb English cucumbers

- Salmon and serving

- ¼ tsp kosher salt

- ¼ tsp pepper

- 1 tbsp olive oil

- Four salmon fillets

- Dill sprigs

Preparation:

1. Mix all the ingredients of the sauce list in a bowl. The sauce is ready. Combine all the items of salad in a bowl and set aside. The salad and dressing are ready.

2. Place fish with skin placed downwards on a baking tray.

3. Grill the fillets for 15 minutes. Place the grilled fillets on a plate and drizzle salad and dressing over it; serve.

Salmon, Lentil & Pomegranate Salad

Prep Time: 15 min

Cook Time: 0 min

Serve: 2

Ingredients:

- One garlic clove chopped

- One red onion sliced

- 1 tsp clear honey

- One pomegranate

- 140 g hot-smoked salmon

- 2 tbsp olive oil

- 2 tbsp chopped tarragon

- 20 g flat-leaf parsley

- 400 g lentil

- juice ½ lemon

- toasted pitta bread, to serve

Preparation:

Combine all the ingredients in a bowl and toss well. Serve and enjoy it.

Salmon and pumpkin salad with chili jam

Prep Time: 30 min

Cook Time: 30 min

Serve: 2

Ingredients:

- lime

- coriander (chopped to serve)

- 700 g pumpkin

- Four salmon fillets

- 200 g green beans

- 125 g baby spinach

- 1 tbsp olive oil

- One sliced Spanish onion

Dressing:

- 2 tbsp lime juice

- 1/2 cup vegetable stock (liquid)

- 1 tbsp fish sauce

- 1 tbsp chili jam

- 1 tbsp brown sugar

Preparation:

1. Combine all the items of dressing in a pan and boil it for few minutes. The dressing is ready. Drizzle oil over pumpkin and roast in a preheated oven at 200 degrees for 25 minutes.

2. Add peas to boiling water and cook for five minutes. Cook salmon in a heated pan for five minutes. Now mix all the items in a bowl and pour dressing.

Salmon with Pomegranate Molasses Glaze

Prep Time: 5 min

Cook Time: 15 min

Serve: 3

Ingredients:

- 1/2 tsp salt

- 1/4 cup pomegranate molasses

- 1/4 tsp cornstarch

- 2 tsp brown sugar

- Four boneless salmon fillets

- Black pepper

- pomegranate seeds for garnish

- Mint for garnishing

Preparation:

1. Whisk pepper, sugar, salt, and starch in a bowl. Coat fillets with the mixture.

2. Fry the fillets in heated oil for five minutes. Transfer the fillets to the baking tray. Drizzle pomegranate molasses over fillets.

3. Bake in a preheated oven at 400 degrees for 15 minutes.

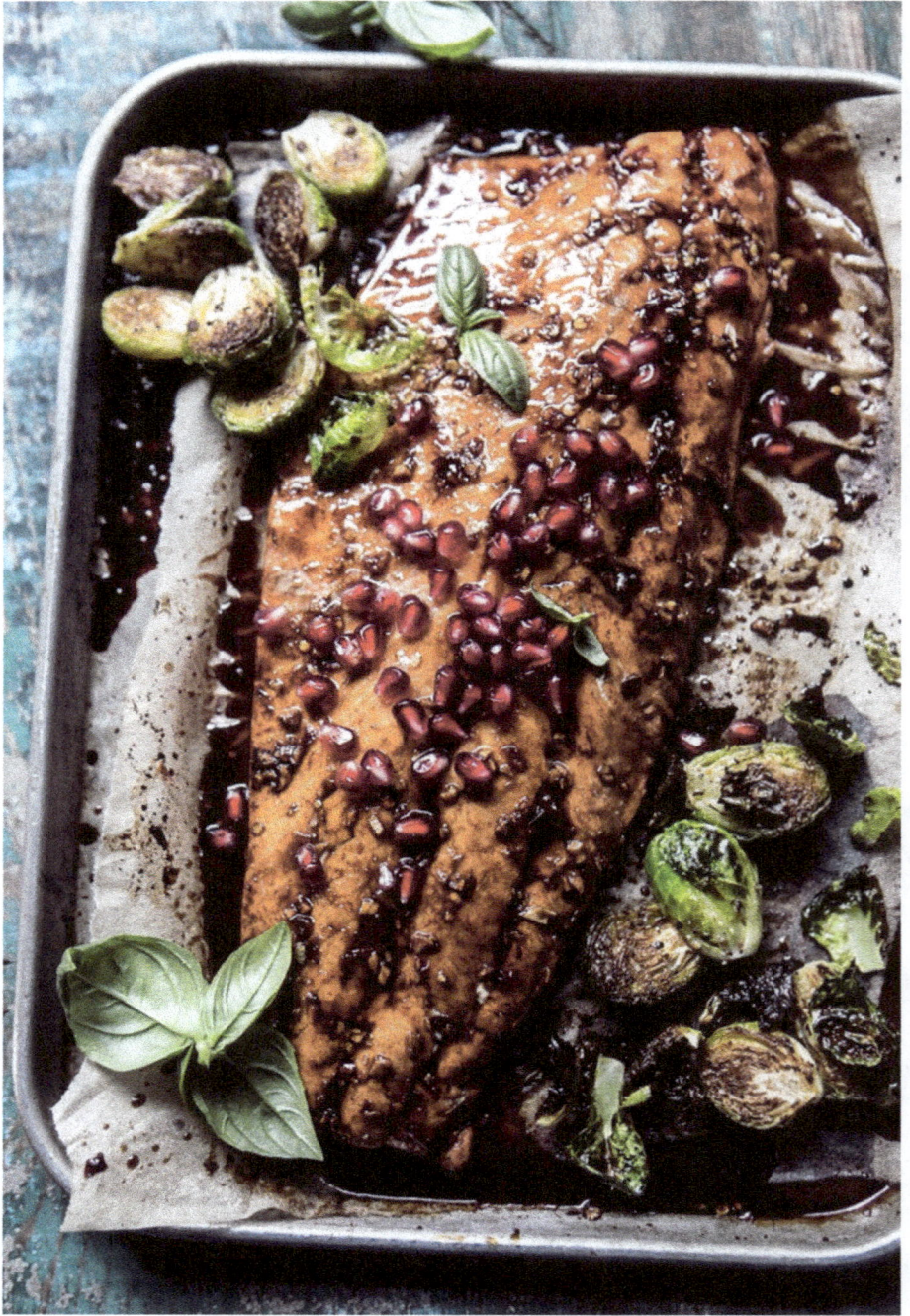

www.ingramcontent.com/pod-product-compliance
Lightning Source LLC
Chambersburg PA
CBHW050752030426
42336CB00012B/1775